FATTY LIVER DIET

COOKBOOK

Delicious Recipes to Heal and Nourish

Your Body

Mary R. Taylor

Table Of Content

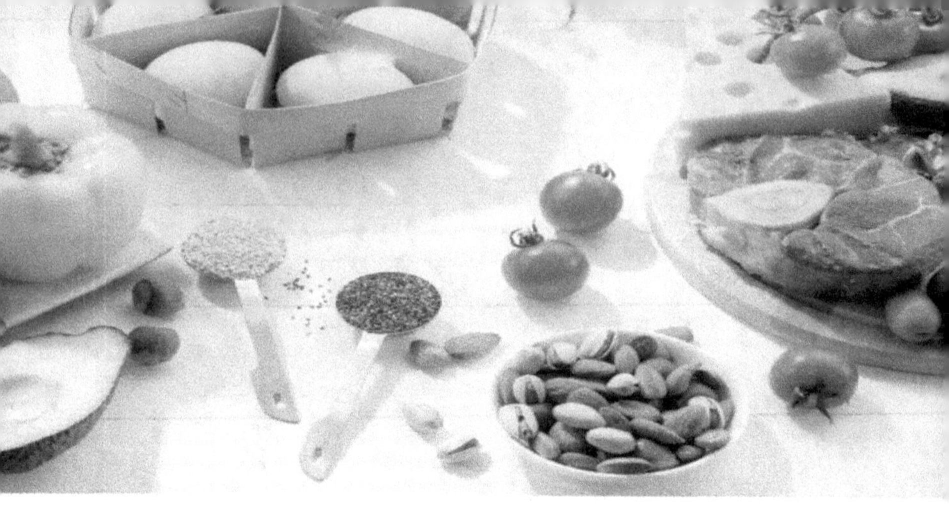

INTRODUCTION

Greetings and welcome to the path to improved general health and liver function. It's likely that you or someone you care about is battling the difficulties associated with fatty liver disease if you've picked up this cookbook. Remember, you're not by yourself. Fatty liver disease is a major health concern in our contemporary culture, affecting millions of people globally and becoming more common.

However, there remains optimism despite the diagnosis and any unknowns that may accompany it. Your fork is one of the most useful instruments you have at your disposal for treating fatty liver disease. Indeed, what you eat has a significant impact on the condition of your liver, and this cookbook will take you on a tasty path to improved liver health.

Understanding Fatty Liver Disease

Even though the word "fatty liver disease" is becoming all too common in today's world, many people still struggle with anxiety and confusion when they hear it. For me, what does that mean? How did that come about? Most importantly, what action can I do to address it? Let's begin with the fundamentals. A deposit of fat in the liver is precisely what is meant to be described as fatty liver disease. Although it was formerly mostly linked to binge drinking, non-alcoholic fatty liver disease (NAFLD) is now the more common type, impacting people of all ages and alcohol consumption levels.

What's most worrisome is that fatty liver disease frequently goes undiagnosed, silently destroying our bodies until symptoms appear or problems develop. And the harm might already be done by then. But here's the thing: power comes from knowledge. The more knowledge we have regarding fatty liver disease, the more capable we are of managing our health and welfare. Now, let us discuss risk factors. Fatty liver disease can arise from a variety of reasons, including obesity, sedentary lifestyles, and poor nutritional choices. The good news is that we can control a large number of these risk factors. We may dramatically lower our risk of fatty liver disease and its related problems by implementing small but effective lifestyle changes, such as eating a healthier diet, exercising more, and controlling our weight.

But knowing that fatty liver disease is not a death sentence is arguably the most liberating part of learning about it. By implementing proactive lifestyle adjustments, early identification, and medical intervention when needed, we can effectively stop the advancement of fatty liver disease and potentially reverse it. Therefore, know that there is hope and that you are not alone if you are struggling with a fatty liver diagnosis. You are able to take charge of your liver health and start along a path to empowerment and wellbeing by educating yourself, making wise decisions, and adopting a proactive attitude toward your wellbeing.

What is Fatty Liver Disease?

The condition known as fatty liver disease is typified by the buildup of fat within the liver cells, which can result in compromised liver function and possible health issues. It includes a wide range of liver diseases, from mild cases like non-alcoholic steatohepatitis (NASH), fibrosis, cirrhosis, and liver cancer, to more serious ones like simple (excessive fat accumulation). Triglycerides build up in liver cells as a result of the liver's impaired capacity to metabolize lipids in fatty liver disease. Alcoholic fatty liver disease (alcoholic fatty liver disease) can be exacerbated by excessive alcohol consumption, but non-alcoholic fatty liver disease (NAFLD) is the most common type and is strongly linked to obesity, insulin resistance, metabolic syndrome, and unhealthy eating patterns.

Although fatty liver disease may not show many symptoms at first, if treatment is not received, the condition may worsen over time without warning signs. It is essential to comprehend the underlying causes and risk factors of fatty liver disease in order to recognize, intervene, and manage the condition early on and provide hope for better liver health and general wellbeing.

Causes and Risk Factors

Triglycerides build up in the liver cells of people with fatty liver disease because the liver's capacity to metabolize fats is compromised. Although alcoholism can be a contributing factor in the development of alcoholic fatty liver disease, non-alcoholic fatty liver disease (NAFLD) has become the most common type and is closely linked to obesity, insulin resistance, metabolic syndrome, and unhealthy eating patterns.

Even while fatty liver disease may not show any signs at first, it can develop gradually and cause major problems if treatment is not received. In order to enhance liver health and general well-being, early detection, intervention, and management of fatty liver disease depend on an understanding of the underlying causes and risk factors of the condition.

Importance of Diet in Managing Fatty Liver

It is impossible to overestimate the impact that nutrition plays in the development and management of fatty liver disease because it is fundamental to both of these processes. In certain situations, a nutritious diet can even help repair liver disease by reducing inflammation in the liver and symptom relief. Reducing dietary factors that lead to the production of liver fat is essential to controlling fatty liver disease. This entails consuming less foods heavy in sugar, trans fats, saturated fats, and refined and processed carbs. Rather, the focus should be on eating full, nutrient-dense foods that promote liver health.

Fruits, vegetables, whole grains, lean proteins, and healthy fats like those in nuts, seeds, and fatty fish are essential elements of a diet that is beneficial to the liver. These foods are high in fiber, vitamins, minerals, and antioxidants that assist liver detoxification processes, lower inflammation, and improve metabolic health in general. Furthermore, controlling weight and lowering liver fat requires careful consideration of portion sizes and total calorie intake. Measures as small as 5–10% of body weight reduction can have a major positive impact on insulin sensitivity and liver health.

Food preparation techniques are important in addition to what to consume. Baking, grilling, steaming, and sautéing are healthy cooking techniques that are favored over frying or deep-frying since they reduce calorie consumption and can introduce bad fats. In addition to particular diets, lifestyle choices including the timing and frequency of meals can also affect liver function. Regularly eating well-balanced meals throughout the day helps control blood sugar levels and keeps the liver from storing too much fat.

In the end, following a liver-friendly diet is about fostering general health and wellbeing, not simply treating fatty liver disease. People may maintain liver function, slow the course of disease, and enhance their overall quality of life by feeding their bodies with nutritious, nutrient-dense meals and developing healthy eating habits.

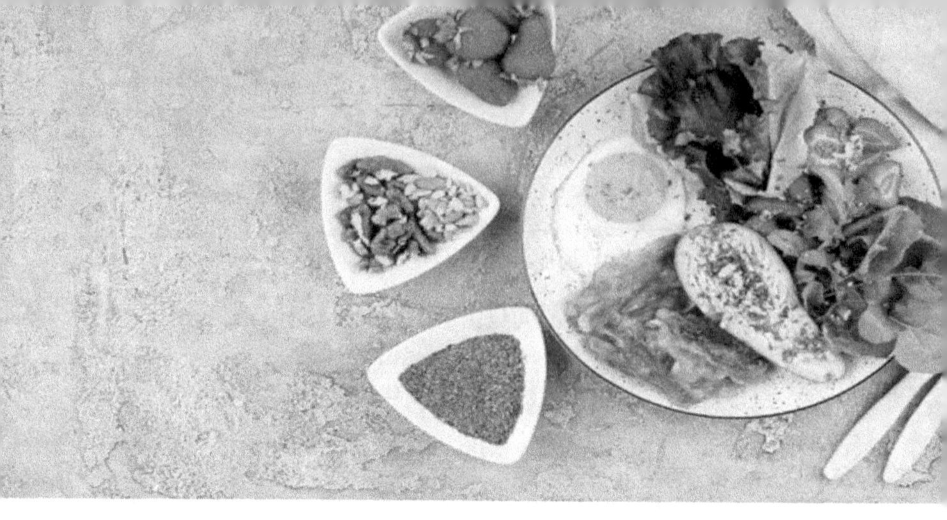

CHAPTER 1: FOUNDATIONS OF A HEALTHY DIET FOR FATTY LIVER

As the foundation of both preventative and treatment plans, nutrition is vital in the management of fatty liver disease. A balanced diet can lower inflammation, support overall liver function, and address the underlying causes of liver fat formation.

Important dietary considerations for managing fatty liver include:

1. Balance of macronutrients: Stressing a diet high in lean proteins, complex carbs, and

healthy fats while limiting intake of processed foods, sweets, and saturated fats helps control blood sugar levels, encourage fullness, and prevent the buildup of liver fat.

2. Micronutrients and Antioxidants: Eating a lot of fruits, vegetables, and whole grains gives you important vitamins, minerals, and antioxidants that help fight inflammation, lessen oxidative stress, and promote liver detoxification processes.

3. Fiber: Foods high in fiber, like fruits, vegetables, legumes, and whole grains, support healthy liver function by facilitating digestion, enhancing sensations of fullness, and assisting in the regulation of cholesterol levels.

4. Hydration: Keeping the body properly hydrated helps the liver function by assisting in the removal of toxins and waste products from metabolism.

5. Portion Control and Moderation: Limiting calories and gaining weight are two things that might make fatty liver disease worse. By using these strategies, you can avoid these problems.

A nutrient-rich diet should be prioritized by those who want to manage fatty liver disease, lower their risk of complications, and enhance their liver's general health and function.

Foods to Limit or Avoid

Being aware of the things we eat is crucial for treating fatty liver disease. Some dietary choices may worsen the illness by aggravating inflammation and hepatic fat storage. To promote liver health, limit or stay away from the following foods:

1. Sugary Foods and Drinks: Sugary foods and drinks, such as cakes, candies, sodas, and sweetened beverages, include a lot of added sugar, which can lead to the development of

liver fat and insulin resistance. Reducing sugar consumption or using natural sweeteners like fruit can help lessen these effects.

2. Processed Foods: Foods high in fats, carbohydrates, and additives that are bad for the liver and cause inflammation, such as fast food, frozen dinners, and prepackaged snacks, are examples of processed foods. Selecting whole, minimally processed foods promotes liver health and gives you more control over the components.

3. heavy-Fat Foods: Foods heavy in trans and saturated fats, like fatty meats, fried foods, and full-fat dairy products, can exacerbate inflammation and lead to the buildup of liver fat. Rather, go for lean protein sources like fish, chicken, and plant-based substitutes, and select healthy fats from foods like olive oil, avocados, and almonds.

People can actively manage fatty liver disease and enhance general liver health by being aware of certain items and making educated dietary decisions.

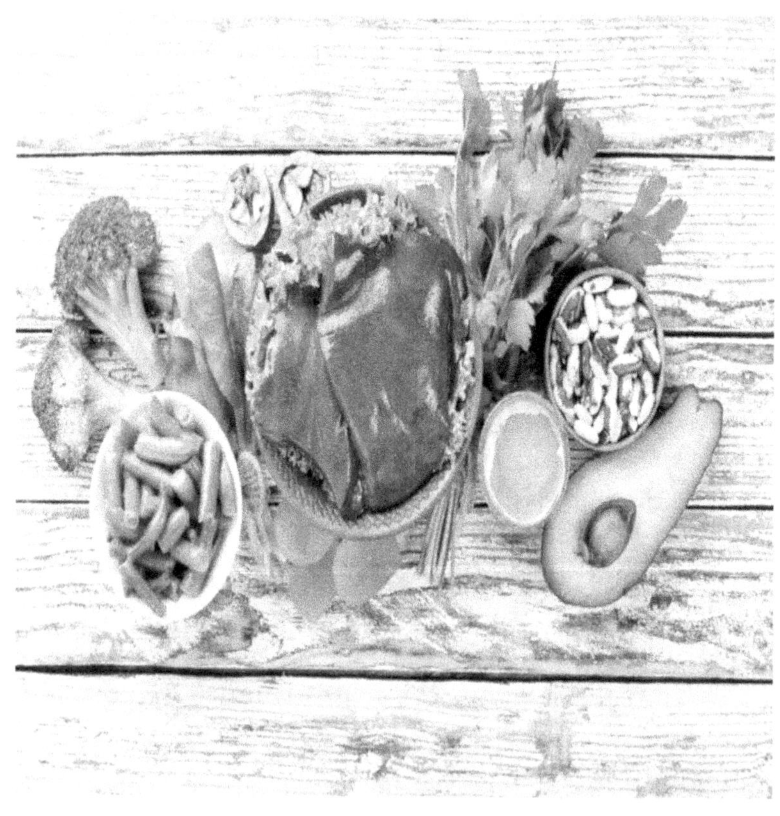

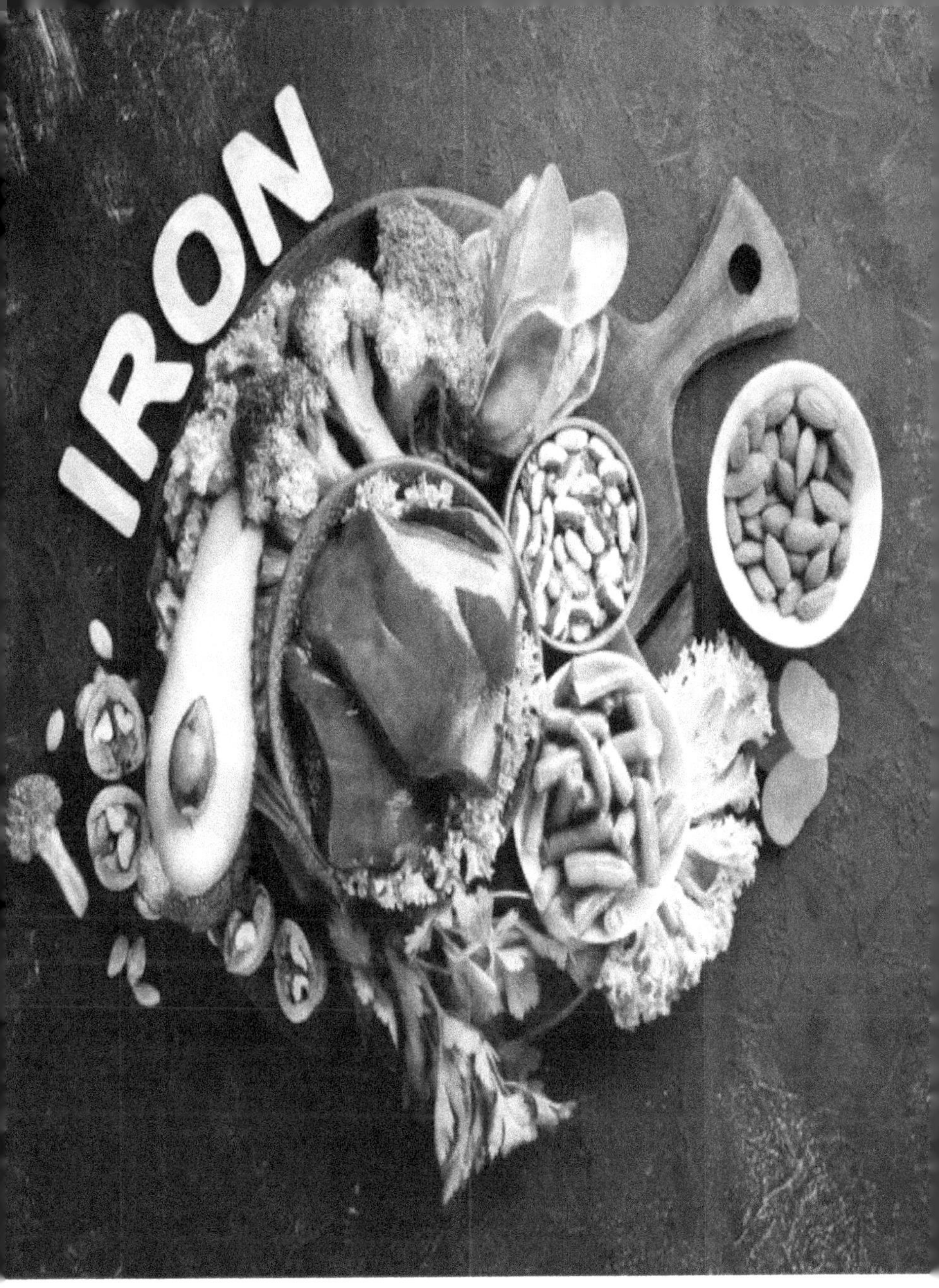
IRON

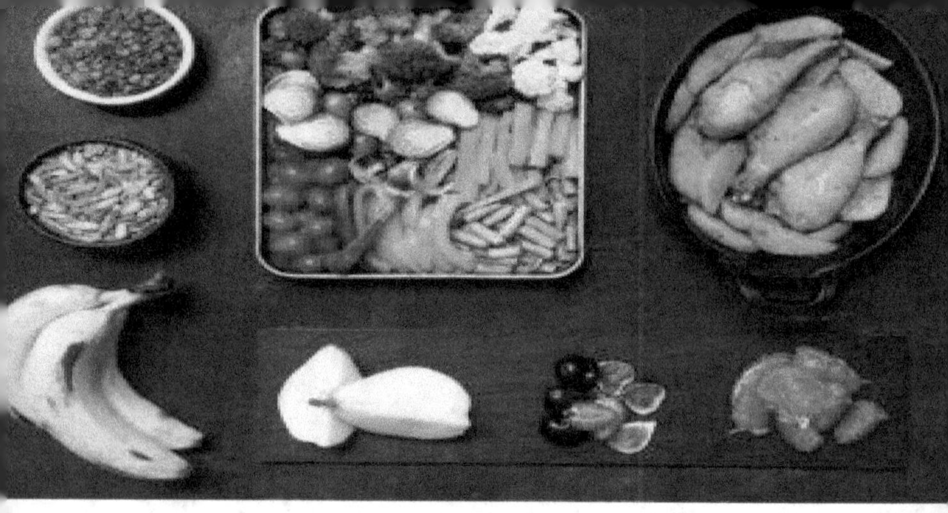

CHAPTER 2: MEAL PLANNING AND PREPARATION TIPS

Developing a Meal Plan for Fatty Liver

Designing a nutritious and well-balanced eating pattern that promotes liver health and lowers inflammation and fat accumulation is the first step in designing a meal plan for fatty liver. Take into consideration these crucial steps:

1. Emphasis on Whole Foods: Create meals that are centered around produce, whole grains, lean meats, healthy fats, and fruits and vegetables that have undergone little

processing. The vital vitamins, minerals, antioxidants, and fiber found in these nutrient-dense foods promote liver function and general health.

2. Place a Focus on Plant-Based Foods: Make sure that all of your meals include a variety of plant-based foods, such as fruits, vegetables, legumes, nuts, seeds, and whole grains. Plant-based diets can help lower inflammation and enhance liver function, and they are linked to lower risks of fatty liver disease.

3. Lean Protein Sources to Consider: Lean protein options include fish, fowl, tofu, tempeh, beans, and lentils. For those with fatty liver disease, these proteins are a better choice because they have less cholesterol and saturated fat than fatty portions of meat.

4. Limit Refined Carbohydrates and Added Sugars: Cut back on sugar-filled foods and drinks, as well as refined carbs found in items

like white rice, bread, and pastries. These foods have the potential to raise blood sugar levels and cause the buildup of liver fat.

5. Control Portion Sizes: To avoid overindulging and consuming too many calories, which can lead to weight gain and the accumulation of liver fat, pay attention to portion sizes and engage in mindful eating.

Following these recommendations and consulting with a physician or qualified dietitian can help people design a customized eating plan that supports liver function and enhances general wellbeing.

Portion Control and Moderation

For the purpose of treating fatty liver disease and enhancing general liver health, portion control and moderation are crucial. Although it can be easy to concentrate only on what meals to consume, quantity is just as essential, particularly when it comes to foods that are high in fat and calories.

Portion sizes have increased for many people over time, which has resulted in weight gain and excessive calorie intake—both of which can worsen fatty liver disease. But exercising portion control does not imply feeling deprived or constrained. It all comes down to striking a balance and consuming food in a way that advances your health objectives.

Start by paying closer attention to portion sizes and your body's signals of hunger and fullness. You may reduce overeating and increase pleasure with fewer portions of food by using smaller plates and bowls, portioning meals appropriately, and avoiding mindless eating.

Additionally, when it comes to decadent or low-nutrient foods, moderation is essential. Treats are fine once in a while, but moderation is key to avoiding overindulging in sugars, bad fats, and empty calories, all of which can lead to the buildup of liver fat. People can take charge of their caloric intake, regulate their weight, and promote liver health by engaging in portion management and moderation practices. Modest but sustained dietary modifications can have a major positive impact on fatty liver disease and general health.

Healthy Cooking Methods

For the purpose of treating fatty liver disease and enhancing liver health, using healthful cooking techniques is essential. People can minimize their consumption of harmful fats and calories while optimizing the benefits of nutrient-rich sources by choosing cooking methods that minimize added fats and maintain the nutritional integrity of foods.

Some healthy cooking techniques to think about are:

1. Baking: Baking eliminates the need for additional fats or oils and allows food to cook evenly. It's a fantastic way to cook nutritious grains, lean meats, and veggies without sacrificing any of their natural nutrients or flavors. Cooking meats, fish, and vegetables

over a grill is a tasty way to prepare food without consuming additional fat. It lets superfluous fats trickle out while adding a smokey flavor and caramelization.

2. Steaming: Steaming is a low-heat cooking technique that keeps food's original flavors, textures, and nutrients. It works especially well with cereals, seafood, and vegetables.

3. Sautéing: Without overpowering food with extra fat, sautéing in a tiny amount of healthful oil, like olive or avocado oil, can provide flavor and richness.

4. Roasting: The natural flavors of vegetables, meats, and tofu are enhanced and a delightful caramelization is produced when they are roasted. It makes meal preparation simple and calls for little additional fat.

Through the use of these healthful cooking techniques, people can expand their culinary skills and enjoy tasty, filling meals that promote liver health and general wellbeing.

Tips for Grocery Shopping and Ingredient Selection

It might be intimidating to navigate the grocery store aisles, particularly if you have fatty liver disease. But with a few easy pointers and strategies, you may choose foods that promote liver health and general wellbeing while making grocery shopping a breeze. Above all, make sure you have a shopping list before you go. Making a list of the materials you'll need and organizing your meals in advance will help you stay focused and prevent you from making impulsive, unhealthy food purchases. Give entire, nutrient-dense foods first priority when choosing ingredients. Consume an abundance of fresh produce, whole grains, lean proteins (fish, poultry, and plant-based options), and healthy fats (avocado, nuts, and seeds). Pay attention to ingredient lists and labels. Select goods with low levels of artificial chemicals, bad fats, and added sugars. When choosing bread, pasta, and cereals, go for whole grains. When choosing dairy products, choose low-fat or fat-free options. Remember the aisles surrounding the fresh vegetables, meats, and dairy products in the supermarket store. The bulk of your shopping basket should consist of these complete foods.

Finally, have no fear of experimenting with new ingredients and recipes. A wide variety of nutrients that support liver function can be found in new fruits, vegetables, grains, and spices that you can try to add excitement and diversity to your meals. You may build a pantry full of foods that fuel your body and help you on your path to improved liver health by using these suggestions and making wise grocery shop selections.

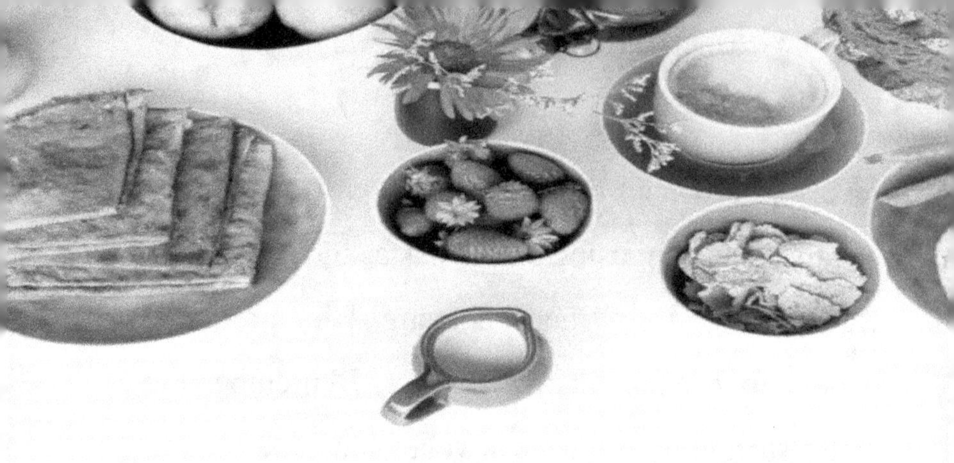

CHAPTER 3: BREAKFAST DELIGHTS FOR LIVER HEALTH

Avocado Toast with Smoked Salmon

Ingredients:

Whole grain bread, ripe avocado, smoked salmon, lemon juice, salt, pepper.

Instructions:

Toast the bread, spread the avocado and lemon juice on it, add the smoked salmon on top, and season with salt & pepper.

:

Rich in omega-3 fatty acids, fiber, and antioxidants.

Nutritional values (per serving)

- ✓ Calories: 300-400
- ✓ Protein: 15-20g
- ✓ Fat: 15-20g
- ✓ Carbohydrates: 25-30g
- ✓ Fiber: 5-8g

Greek Yogurt Parfait

Ingredients:

Greek yogurt, mixed berries, honey, granola.

Instructions:

In a glass or dish, arrange Greek yogurt, granola, and mixed berries; sprinkle with honey.

Nutrients:

High in protein, probiotics, antioxidants, and fiber.

Nutritional values (per serving)

- ✓ Calories: 250-350
- ✓ Protein: 15-20g
- ✓ Fat: 5-10g
- ✓ Carbohydrates: 30-40g
- ✓ Fiber: 5-8g

Spinach and Mushroom Omelette

Ingredients:

Eggs, spinach, mushrooms, onion, garlic, olive oil, salt, pepper.

Instructions:

Add the sliced mushrooms and spinach after sautéing the chopped onion and garlic in olive oil until the spinach wilts. Whisk eggs, add to vegetables, and simmer until solid.

Nutrients:

Packed with protein, vitamins A, C, and K, folate, and antioxidants.

Nutritional values (per serving)

- ✓ Calories: 250-350
- ✓ Protein: 15-20g
- ✓ Fat: 15-20g
- ✓ Carbohydrates: 5-10g
- ✓ Fiber: 2-4g

Quinoa Breakfast Bowl

Ingredients:

Cooked quinoa, almond milk, banana slices, almond butter, cinnamon, honey.

Instructions:

Warm up the cooked quinoa with almond milk, then garnish with almond butter, banana pieces, honey, cinnamon, and a drizzle.

Nutrients:

High in protein, fiber, vitamins, and minerals.

Nutritional values (per serving)

- ✓ Calories: 300-400

- ✓ Protein: 10-15g
- ✓ Fat: 10-15g
- ✓ Carbohydrates: 40-50g
- ✓ Fiber: 5-8g

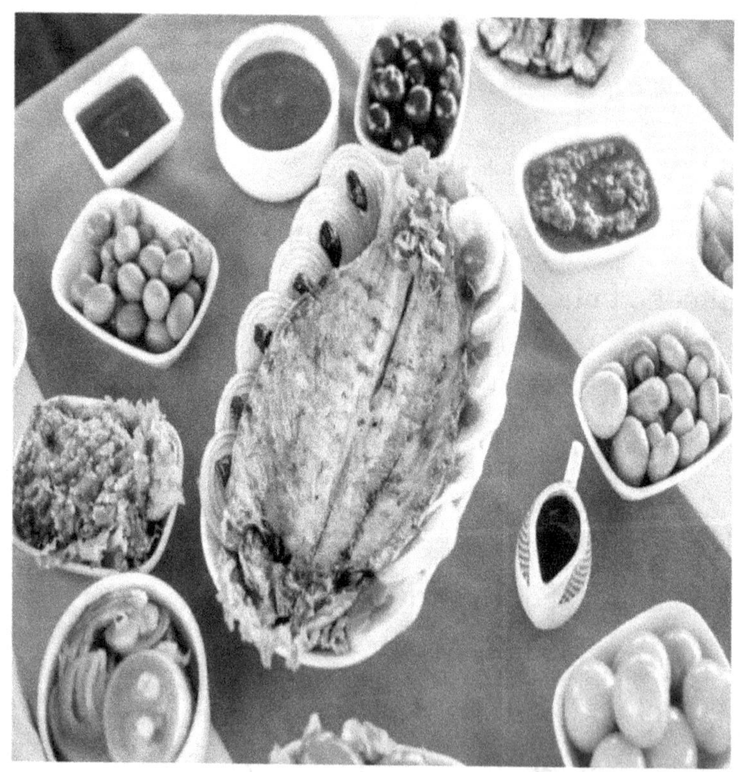

Chia Seed Pudding

Ingredients:

Chia seeds, almond milk, vanilla extract, maple syrup, mixed berries.

Instructions:

Chia seeds should be combined with almond milk, maple syrup, and vanilla essence and left overnight. Garnish with a mixture of berries..

Nutrients:

Rich in omega-3 fatty acids, fiber, protein, and antioxidants.

Nutritional values (per serving)

- ✓ Calories: 200-300
- ✓ Protein: 5-10g
- ✓ Fat: 10-15g
- ✓ Carbohydrates: 20-30g
- ✓ Fiber: 10-15g

Sweet Potato Breakfast Hash

Ingredients:

Sweet potatoes, bell peppers, onion, garlic, olive oil, smoked paprika, salt, pepper, eggs.

Instructions:

Diced sweet potatoes, bell peppers, and onion should be sautéed till soft in olive oil together with garlic and smoky paprika. Top with cooked eggs and serve.

Nutrients:

High in fiber, vitamins A and C, potassium, and antioxidants.

Nutritional values (per serving)

- ✓ Calories: 300-400
- ✓ Protein: 5-10g
- ✓ Fat: 10-15g
- ✓ Carbohydrates: 40-50g
- ✓ Fiber: 5-8g

Oatmeal with Walnuts and Berries

Ingredients:

Rolled oats, water or milk, walnuts, mixed berries, honey.

Instructions:

Cook the rolled oats in milk or water, then sprinkle chopped walnuts, mixed berries, and honey on top.

Nutrients:

Rich in fiber, protein, omega-3 fatty acids, antioxidants, and vitamins.

Nutritional values (per serving)

- ✓ Calories: 250-350
- ✓ Protein: 5-10g
- ✓ Fat: 10-15g
- ✓ Carbohydrates: 30-40g
- ✓ Fiber: 5-8g

Egg and Veggie Breakfast Burrito

Ingredients:

Whole grain tortilla, eggs, bell peppers, onion, spinach, avocado, salsa.

Instructions:

Add diced bell peppers, onion, and spinach to scrambled eggs. Roll up tortilla after stuffing it with salsa, sliced avocado, and scrambled eggs.

Nutrients:

High in protein, fiber, vitamins, and minerals.

Nutritional values (per serving)

- ✓ Calories: 300-400
- ✓ Protein: 15-20g
- ✓ Fat: 10-15g
- ✓ Carbohydrates: 30-40g
- ✓ Fiber: 5-8g

Salmon and Spinach Breakfast Wrap

Whole grain wrap, smoked salmon, cream cheese, baby spinach, cucumber.

Spread smoked salmon, baby spinach, cucumber slices, and cream cheese onto a whole grain wrapper. Roll.

Rich in omega-3 fatty acids, protein, vitamins, and antioxidants.

Nutritional values (per serving)

- ✓ Calories: 300-400
- ✓ Protein: 15-20g
- ✓ Fat: 15-20g
- ✓ Carbohydrates: 20-30g
- ✓ Fiber: 5-8g

Green Smoothie

Ingredients:

Spinach, kale, banana, pineapple, almond milk, chia seeds.

Instructions:

Smoothly blend spinach, kale, chia seeds, banana, pineapple, and almond milk.

Nutrients:

Packed with fiber, vitamins, minerals, antioxidants, and omega-3 fatty acids.

Nutritional values (per serving)

- ✓ Calories: 200-300
- ✓ Protein: 5-10g
- ✓ Fat: 5-10g
- ✓ Carbohydrates: 30-40g
- ✓ Fiber: 5-8g

Cottage Cheese and Fruit Bowl

Cottage cheese, mixed fruit (such as berries, kiwi, and mango), almonds, honey.

Present cottage cheese with chopped nuts, assorted fruit, and honey drizzled on top.

High in protein, calcium, vitamins, and antioxidants.

- ✓ Calories: 200-300
- ✓ Protein: 15-20g
- ✓ Fat: 5-10g
- ✓ Carbohydrates: 20-30g
- ✓ Fiber: 3-6g

Whole Grain Pancakes with Berries

Ingredients:

Whole grain pancake mix, almond milk, mixed berries, maple syrup.

Instructions:

Cook the whole grain pancake mix with almond milk, top with maple syrup and mixed berries, and serve.

Nutrients:

Rich in fiber, protein, vitamins, and antioxidants.

Nutritional values (per serving)

- ✓ Calories: 300-400
- ✓ Protein: 5-10g
- ✓ Fat: 5-10g
- ✓ Carbohydrates: 40-50g
- ✓ Fiber: 5-8g

Egg White Veggie Frittata

Ingredients:

Egg whites, bell peppers, onion, spinach, tomatoes, feta cheese, olive oil, salt, pepper.

Instructions:

In a pan with olive oil, sauté chopped bell peppers, onions, spinach, and tomatoes. Add egg whites, sprinkle with feta cheese, and simmer until just set.

Nutrients:

High in protein, vitamins, minerals, and antioxidants.

Nutritional values (per serving)

- ✓ Calories: 200-300
- ✓ Protein: 15-20g
- ✓ Fat: 5-10g
- ✓ Carbohydrates: 10-15g
- ✓ Fiber: 2-4g

Whole Grain Toast with Ricotta and Berries

Ingredients:

Whole grain bread, ricotta cheese, mixed berries, honey.

Instructions:

Spread ricotta cheese on toasted whole grain bread, add mixed berries on top, and sprinkle with honey.

Nutrients:

Rich in protein, fiber, vitamins, and antioxidants.

Nutritional values (per serving)

- ✓ Calories: 200-300
- ✓ Protein: 10-15g
- ✓ Fat: 5-10g
- ✓ Carbohydrates: 20-30g
- ✓ Fiber: 3-6g

Mango Coconut Chia Pudding

Ingredients:

Chia seeds, coconut milk, ripe mango, shredded coconut, honey.

Instructions:

Combine chia seeds, coconut milk, honey, chopped mango, and shredded coconut; refrigerate overnight. Present cold.

Nutrients:

High in omega-3 fatty acids, fiber, vitamins, and antioxidants.

Nutritional values (per serving)

- ✓ Calories: 250-350
- ✓ Protein: 5-10g
- ✓ Fat: 15-20g
- ✓ Carbohydrates: 25-30g
- ✓ Fiber: 10-15g

These tasty and simple-to-make breakfast options also include a range of nutrients to help liver function. Adapt ingredient and portion proportions to each person's unique nutritional requirements and dietary choices.

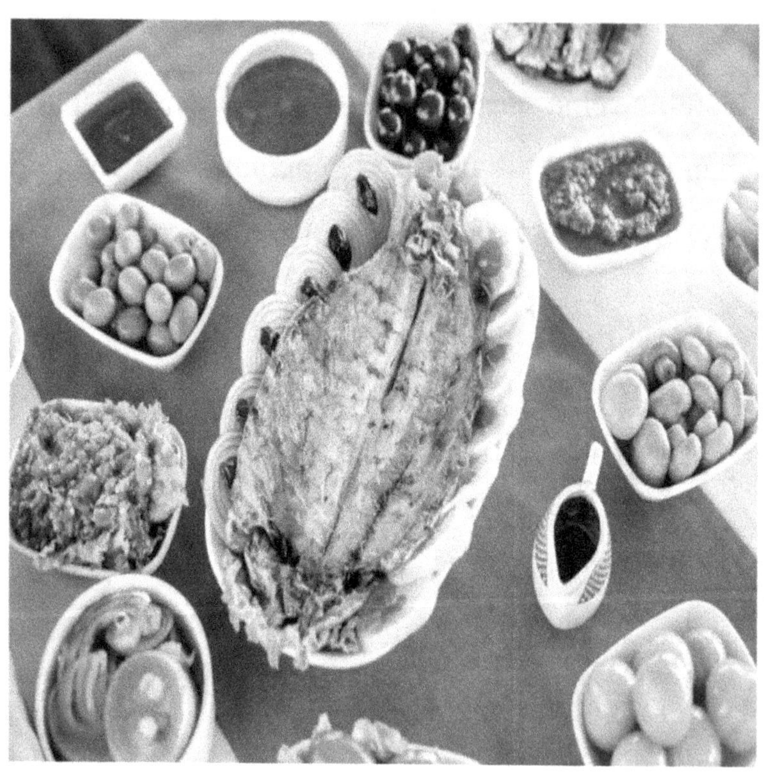

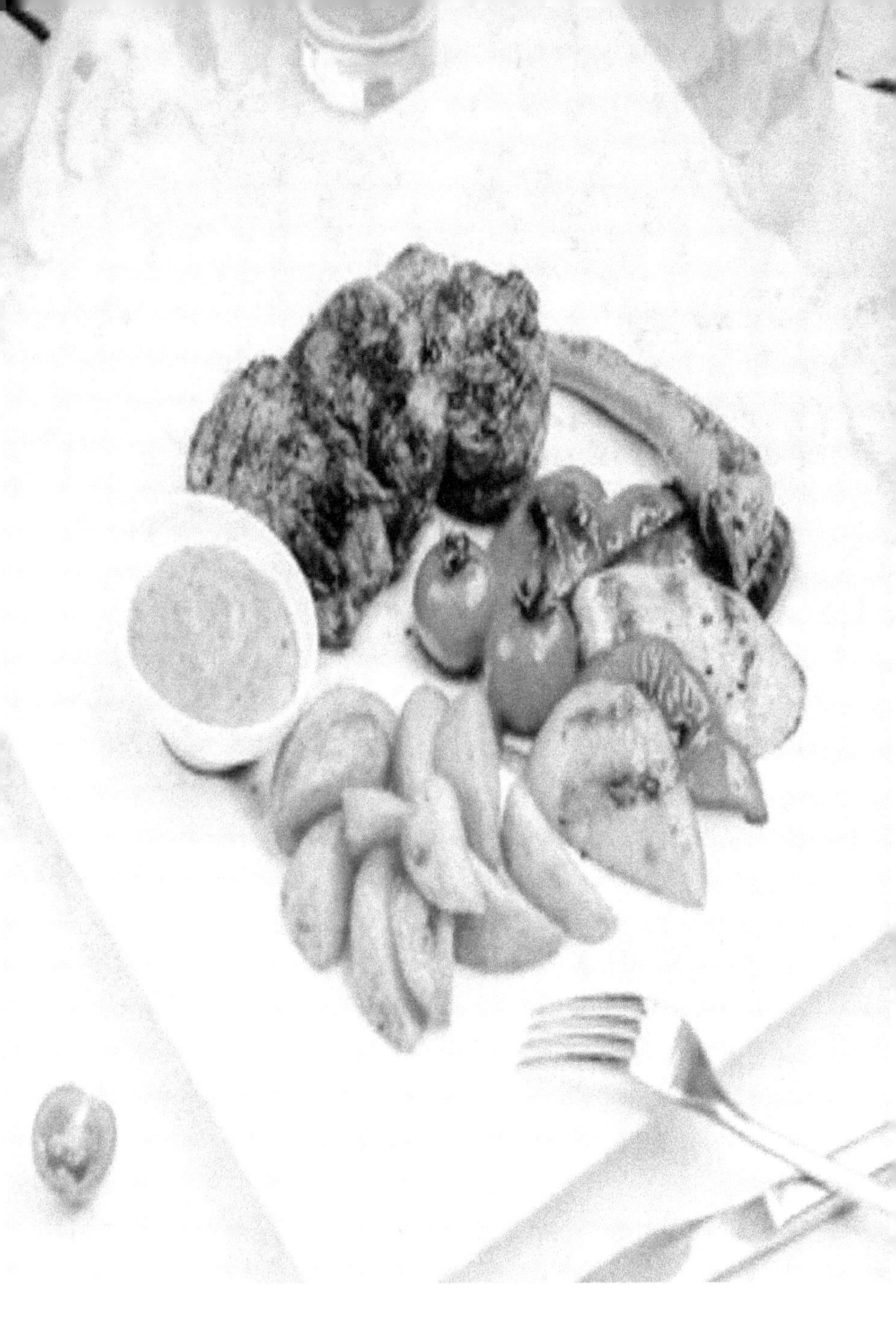

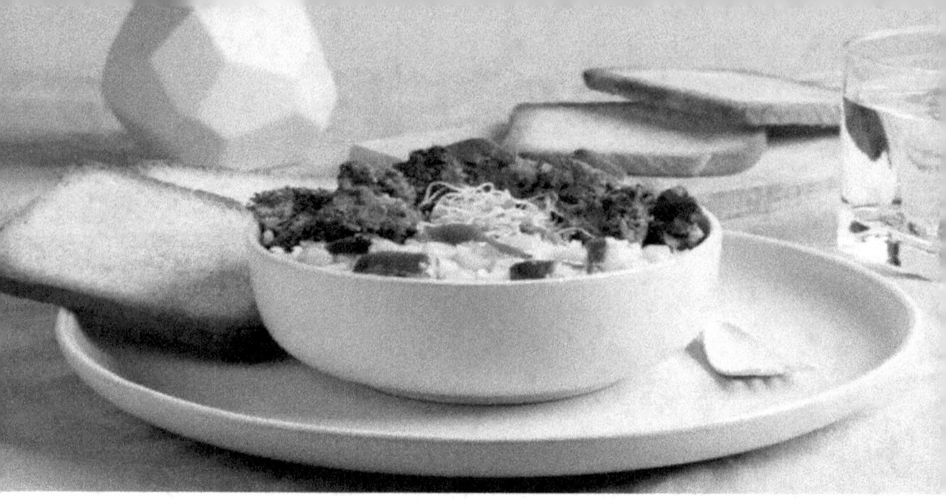

CHAPTER 4: SATISFYING LUNCHES TO SUPPORT LIVER FUNCTION

Grilled Salmon Salad

Ingredients:

Grilled salmon fillet, mixed greens, cherry tomatoes, cucumber, avocado, olive oil, lemon juice, salt, pepper.

Instructions:

Toss mixed greens, cherry tomatoes, cucumber, and avocado with olive oil, lemon juice, salt, and pepper. Top with grilled salmon.

High in omega-3 fatty acids, protein, fiber, vitamins, and antioxidants.

Nutritional values (per serving)

- ✓ Calories: 350-450
- ✓ Protein: 25-30g
- ✓ Fat: 20-25g
- ✓ Carbohydrates: 15-20g
- ✓ Fiber: 5-8g

Quinoa and Black Bean Bowl

Ingredients:

Cooked quinoa, black beans, roasted sweet potatoes, diced bell peppers, corn, avocado, salsa, lime juice, cilantro.

Instructions:

Combine cooked quinoa, black beans, roasted sweet potatoes, diced bell peppers, corn, and avocado. Drizzle with salsa, lime juice, and garnish with cilantro.

Nutrients:

Rich in protein, fiber, vitamins, minerals, and antioxidants.

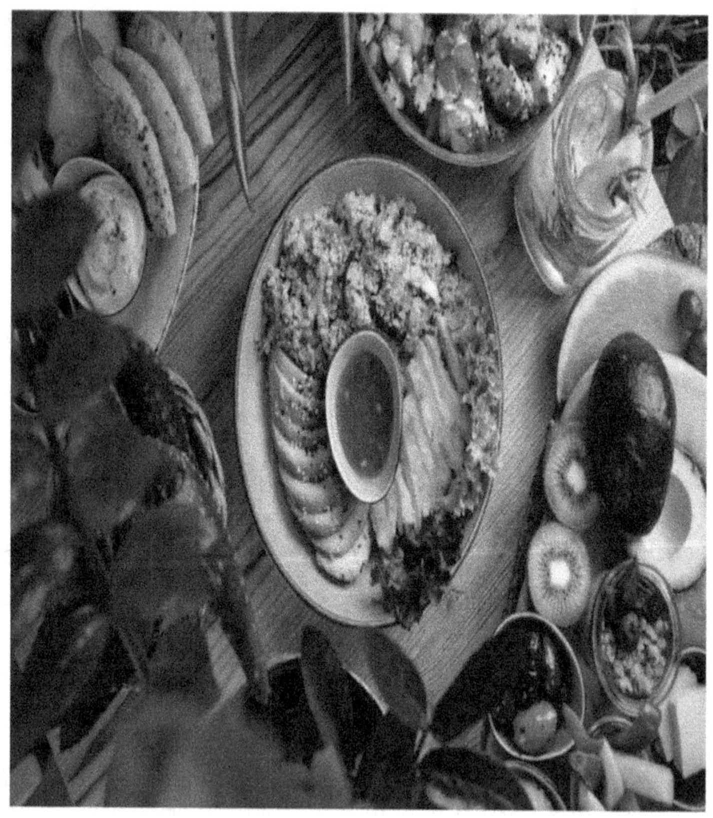

- ✓ Calories: 400-500
- ✓ Protein: 15-20g
- ✓ Fat: 10-15g
- ✓ Carbohydrates: 60-70g
- ✓ Fiber: 10-15g

Turkey and Veggie Wrap

Ingredients:

Whole grain wrap, sliced turkey breast, hummus, spinach, shredded carrots, cucumber, red onion, feta cheese.

Instructions:

Spread hummus on a whole grain wrap, layer with sliced turkey breast, spinach, shredded carrots, cucumber, red onion, and feta cheese. Roll up tightly.

Nutrients:

High in protein, fiber, vitamins, and minerals.

- ✓ Calories: 350-450
- ✓ Protein: 20-25g
- ✓ Fat: 15-20g
- ✓ Carbohydrates: 30-40g
- ✓ Fiber: 5-8g

Stir-Fried Tofu with Vegetables

Ingredients:

Firm tofu, broccoli, bell peppers, snap peas, carrots, garlic, ginger, soy sauce, sesame oil.

Instructions:

Stir-fry cubed tofu with broccoli, bell peppers, snap peas, carrots, garlic, and ginger in soy sauce and sesame oil until vegetables are tender.

Nutrients:

Protein-rich, high in fiber, vitamins, minerals, and antioxidants.

- ✓ Calories: 300-400
- ✓ Protein: 15-20g
- ✓ Fat: 15-20g
- ✓ Carbohydrates: 25-30g
- ✓ Fiber: 5-8g

Mediterranean Chickpea Salad

Ingredients:

Chickpeas, cherry tomatoes, cucumber, red onion, Kalamata olives, feta cheese, olive oil, lemon juice, oregano.

Instructions:

Combine chickpeas, cherry tomatoes, cucumber, red onion, Kalamata olives, and feta cheese. Dress with olive oil, lemon juice, and oregano.

Nutrients:

High in protein, fiber, vitamins, minerals, and healthy fats.

Nutritional values (per serving)

- ✓ Calories: 300-400
- ✓ Protein: 10-15g
- ✓ Fat: 15-20g
- ✓ Carbohydrates: 30-40g
- ✓ Fiber: 10-15g

Vegetable and Lentil Soup

Ingredients:

Lentils, carrots, celery, onion, garlic, vegetable broth, diced tomatoes, spinach, thyme, bay leaf.

Instructions:

Sauté chopped carrots, celery, onion, and garlic until softened. Add lentils, vegetable broth, diced tomatoes, spinach, thyme, and bay leaf. Simmer until lentils are tender.

Nutrients:

High in protein, fiber, vitamins, minerals, and antioxidants.

Nutritional values (per serving)

- ✓ Calories: 250-350
- ✓ Protein: 10-15g
- ✓ Fat: 5-10g
- ✓ Carbohydrates: 40-50g
- ✓ Fiber: 10-15g

Grilled Chicken Caesar Salad

Ingredients:

Grilled chicken breast, romaine lettuce, cherry tomatoes, Parmesan cheese, whole grain croutons, Caesar dressing.

Instructions:

Toss chopped romaine lettuce with cherry tomatoes, grated Parmesan cheese, whole grain croutons, and grilled chicken breast. Drizzle with Caesar dressing.

Nutrients:

High in protein, fiber, vitamins, and minerals.

- ✓ Calories: 400-500
- ✓ Protein: 25-30g
- ✓ Fat: 20-25g
- ✓ Carbohydrates: 15-20g
- ✓ Fiber: 5-8g

Veggie Sushi Rolls

Ingredients:

Sushi rice, nori sheets, cucumber, avocado, carrot, bell pepper, tofu, soy sauce, wasabi, pickled ginger.

Instructions:

Spread sushi rice on nori sheets, add sliced cucumber, avocado, carrot, bell pepper, and tofu. Roll tightly, slice, and serve with soy sauce, wasabi, and pickled ginger.

Nutrients:

Protein-rich, high in fiber, vitamins, minerals, and antioxidants.

- ✓ Calories: 300-400
- ✓ Protein: 10-15g
- ✓ Fat: 5-10g
- ✓ Carbohydrates: 50-60g
- ✓ Fiber: 5-8g

Shrimp and Vegetable Stir-Fry

Ingredients:

Shrimp, bell peppers, snap peas, broccoli, carrots, garlic, ginger, soy sauce, honey, sesame oil.

Instructions:

Stir-fry shrimp with sliced bell peppers, snap peas, broccoli, carrots, garlic, and ginger in soy sauce, honey, and sesame oil until cooked through.

Nutrients:

Protein-rich, high in fiber, vitamins, minerals, and antioxidants.

- ✓ Calories: 300-400
- ✓ Protein: 20-25g
- ✓ Fat: 10-15g
- ✓ Carbohydrates: 20-25g
- ✓ Fiber: 5-8g

Tuna Salad Stuffed Avocado

Ingredients:

Canned tuna, avocado, cherry tomatoes, red onion, cucumber, lemon juice, olive oil, salt, pepper.

Instructions:

Mix canned tuna with diced cherry tomatoes, red onion, cucumber, lemon juice, olive oil, salt, and pepper. Serve stuffed into halved avocados.

Nutrients:

High in protein, fiber, healthy fats, vitamins, and minerals.

- ✓ Calories: 300-400
- ✓ Protein: 15-20g
- ✓ Fat: 20-25g
- ✓ Carbohydrates: 10-15g
- ✓ Fiber: 8-12g

Turkey and Veggie Quinoa Bowl

Ingredients:

Cooked quinoa, sliced turkey breast, roasted vegetables (such as sweet potatoes, Brussels sprouts, and cauliflower), spinach, cranberries, almonds, balsamic vinaigrette.

Instructions:

Combine cooked quinoa, sliced turkey breast, roasted vegetables, spinach, cranberries, and almonds. Drizzle with balsamic vinaigrette.

Nutrients:

Protein-rich, high in fiber, vitamins, minerals, and antioxidants.

Nutritional values (per serving)

- ✓ Calories: 400-500
- ✓ Protein: 25-30g
- ✓ Fat: 15-20g
- ✓ Carbohydrates: 40-50g
- ✓ Fiber: 8-12g

Chickpea and Avocado Salad

Ingredients:

Chickpeas, avocado, cherry tomatoes, cucumber, red onion, feta cheese, olive oil, lemon juice, parsley.

Instructions:

Mix chickpeas with diced avocado, cherry tomatoes, cucumber, red onion, feta cheese, olive oil, lemon juice, and parsley.

Nutrients:

High in protein, fiber, healthy fats, vitamins, minerals, and antioxidants.

Nutritional values (per serving)

- ✓ Calories: 350-450
- ✓ Protein: 10-15g
- ✓ Fat: 20-25g
- ✓ Carbohydrates: 30-40g
- ✓ Fiber: 10-15g

Eggplant and Lentil Curry

Ingredients:

Eggplant, lentils, onion, garlic, ginger, tomatoes, coconut milk, curry powder, cilantro.

Instructions:

Sauté diced eggplant, onion, garlic, and ginger until softened. Add cooked lentils, diced tomatoes, coconut milk, and curry powder. Simmer until flavors meld. Garnish with cilantro.

Protein-rich, high in fiber, vitamins, minerals, and antioxidants.

Nutritional values (per serving)

- ✓ Calories: 300-400
- ✓ Protein: 15-20g
- ✓ Fat: 10-15g
- ✓ Carbohydrates: 40-50g
- ✓ Fiber: 10-15g

Chicken and Vegetable Lettuce Wraps

Ingredients:

Ground chicken, lettuce leaves, bell peppers, water chestnuts, green onions, garlic, ginger, soy sauce, hoisin sauce.

Instructions:

Stir-fry ground chicken with sliced bell peppers, chopped water chestnuts, green onions, garlic, and ginger in soy sauce and hoisin sauce. Serve in lettuce leaves.

Protein-rich, high in fiber, vitamins, minerals, and antioxidants.

- ✓ Calories: 300-400
- ✓ Protein: 20-25g
- ✓ Fat: 10-15g
- ✓ Carbohydrates: 20-25g
- ✓ Fiber: 5-8g

Salmon and Asparagus Foil Packets

Salmon fillets, asparagus spears, cherry tomatoes, lemon slices, olive oil, garlic, dill, salt, pepper.

Place salmon fillets on foil, surround with asparagus spears, cherry tomatoes, and lemon slices. Drizzle with olive oil, minced garlic, chopped dill, salt, and pepper. Seal foil packets and bake until salmon is cooked through.

High in omega-3 fatty acids, protein, fiber, vitamins, and antioxidants.

- ✓ Calories: 350-450
- ✓ Protein: 25-30g
- ✓ Fat: 15-20g
- ✓ Carbohydrates: 10-15g
- ✓ Fiber: 5-8g

As you explore the recipes and insights within this cookbook, I kindly request a moment of your time. Your review on Amazon would greatly assist others on their journey to better liver health. Whether you found the recipes delicious, the nutritional tips valuable, or simply enjoyed the read, your feedback is invaluable. Thank you for considering sharing your thoughts and for being a part of spreading awareness about the importance of a healthy liver and balanced nutrition.

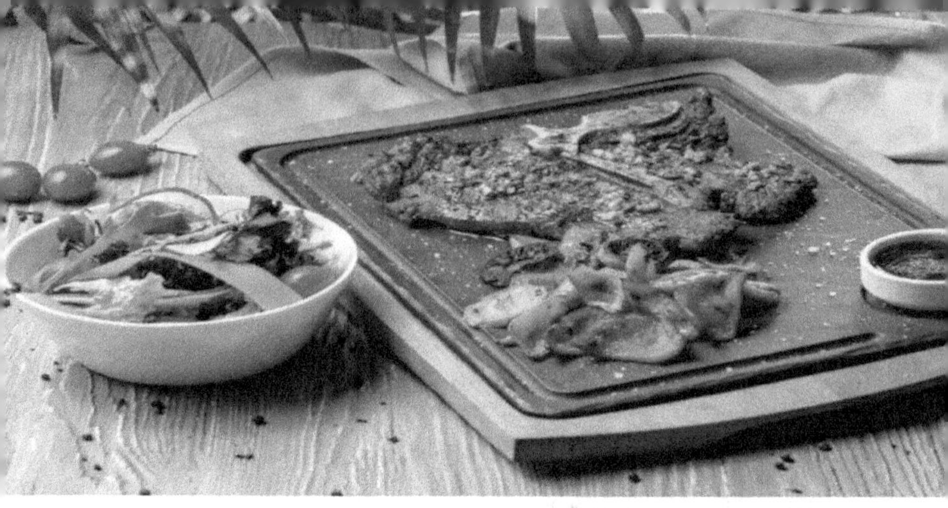

CHAPTER 5: NOURISHING DINNERS FOR LIVER WELLNESS

Grilled Salmon with Roasted Vegetables

Ingredients:

Salmon fillets, sweet potatoes, Brussels sprouts, carrots, olive oil, garlic powder, salt, pepper.

Instructions:

Season salmon with garlic powder, salt, and pepper. Roast sweet potatoes, Brussels sprouts, and carrots tossed in olive oil, salt, and pepper. Grill salmon until cooked through. Serve with roasted vegetables.

High in omega-3 fatty acids, protein, fiber, vitamins, and antioxidants.

- ✓ Calories: 400-500
- ✓ Protein: 25-30g
- ✓ Fat: 20-25g
- ✓ Carbohydrates: 20-25g
- ✓ Fiber: 5-8g

Turkey and Vegetable Stir-Fry

Ground turkey, broccoli, bell peppers, snap peas, carrots, garlic, ginger, soy sauce, sesame oil.

Stir-fry ground turkey with chopped broccoli, bell peppers, snap peas, carrots, garlic, and ginger in soy sauce and sesame oil until turkey is cooked through and vegetables are tender.

Nutrients:

High in protein, fiber, vitamins, minerals, and antioxidants.

Nutritional values (per serving)

- ✓ Calories: 350-450
- ✓ Protein: 25-30g
- ✓ Fat: 15-20g
- ✓ Carbohydrates: 20-25g
- ✓ Fiber: 5-8g

Baked Chicken Breast with Quinoa and Steamed Greens

Ingredients:

Chicken breast, quinoa, spinach, kale, lemon, olive oil, garlic, salt, pepper.

Season chicken breast with salt, pepper, and lemon juice. Bake until cooked through. Cook quinoa according to package instructions. Steam spinach and kale. Serve chicken with quinoa and steamed greens.

Nutrients:

Protein-rich, high in fiber, vitamins, minerals, and antioxidants.

Nutritional values (per serving)

- ✓ Calories: 400-500
- ✓ Protein: 25-30g
- ✓ Fat: 10-15g
- ✓ Carbohydrates: 30-35g
- ✓ Fiber: 5-8g

Vegetarian Lentil Soup

Ingredients:

Lentils, onion, carrots, celery, garlic, vegetable broth, diced tomatoes, spinach, cumin, turmeric, salt, pepper.

Instructions:

Sauté chopped onion, carrots, celery, and garlic until softened. Add lentils, vegetable broth, diced tomatoes, cumin, turmeric, salt, and pepper. Simmer until lentils are tender. Stir in spinach before serving.

Nutrients:

High in protein, fiber, vitamins, minerals, and antioxidants.

Nutritional values (per serving)

- ✓ Calories: 300-400
- ✓ Protein: 15-20g
- ✓ Fat: 5-10g

- ✓ Carbohydrates: 40-50g
- ✓ Fiber: 15-20g

Salmon and Vegetable Foil Packets

Ingredients:

Salmon fillets, zucchini, bell peppers, cherry tomatoes, lemon, olive oil, garlic, dill, salt, pepper.

Instructions:

Place salmon fillets on foil, surround with sliced zucchini, bell peppers, cherry tomatoes, lemon slices, minced garlic, chopped dill, salt, and pepper. Seal foil packets and bake until salmon is cooked through.

Nutrients:

Rich in omega-3 fatty acids, protein, fiber, vitamins, and antioxidants.

Nutritional values (per serving)

- ✓ Calories: 350-450
- ✓ Protein: 25-30g

- ✓ Fat: 15-20g
- ✓ Carbohydrates: 10-15g
- ✓ Fiber: 5-8g

Grilled Chicken Caesar Salad

Ingredients:

Grilled chicken breast, romaine lettuce, cherry tomatoes, Parmesan cheese, whole grain croutons, Caesar dressing.

Instructions:

Toss chopped romaine lettuce with cherry tomatoes, grated Parmesan cheese, whole grain croutons, and grilled chicken breast. Drizzle with Caesar dressing.

Nutrients:

High in protein, fiber, vitamins, and minerals.

Nutritional values (per serving)

- ✓ Calories: 350-450
- ✓ Protein: 25-30g

- ✓ Fat: 15-20g
- ✓ Carbohydrates: 15-20g
- ✓ Fiber: 5-8g

Vegetable and Tofu Stir-Fry

Ingredients:

Firm tofu, broccoli, bell peppers, snap peas, carrots, onion, garlic, ginger, soy sauce, sesame oil.

Instructions:

Stir-fry cubed tofu with chopped broccoli, bell peppers, snap peas, carrots, onion, garlic, and ginger in soy sauce and sesame oil until vegetables are tender.

Nutrients:

Protein-rich, high in fiber, vitamins, minerals, and antioxidants.

- ✓ Calories: 300-400

- ✓ Protein: 15-20g

- ✓ Fat: 15-20g

- ✓ Carbohydrates: 20-25g

- ✓ Fiber: 5-8g

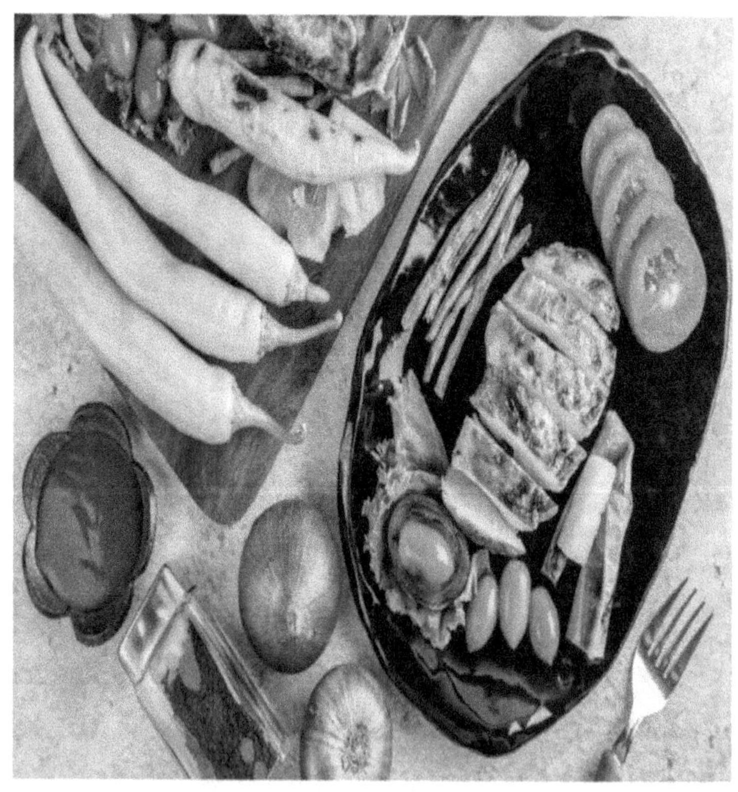

Baked Cod with Roasted Vegetables

Ingredients:

Cod fillets, cauliflower, asparagus, cherry tomatoes, lemon, olive oil, garlic, thyme, salt, pepper.

Instructions:

Season cod fillets with olive oil, minced garlic, thyme, salt, and pepper. Roast cauliflower, asparagus, and cherry tomatoes tossed in olive oil, salt, and pepper. Bake cod until cooked through. Serve with roasted vegetables.

Nutrients:

High in protein, fiber, vitamins, and antioxidants.

Nutritional values (per serving)

- ✓ Calories: 300-400
- ✓ Protein: 25-30g
- ✓ Fat: 10-15g
- ✓ Carbohydrates: 20-25g

✓ Fiber: 5-8g

Chickpea and Spinach Curry

Ingredients:

Chickpeas, spinach, onion, garlic, ginger, tomatoes, coconut milk, curry powder, turmeric, cumin, coriander, salt, pepper.

Instructions:

Sauté chopped onion, garlic, and ginger until softened. Add chickpeas, diced tomatoes, coconut milk, curry powder, turmeric, cumin, coriander, salt, and pepper. Simmer until flavors meld. Stir in spinach before serving.

Nutrients:

Protein-rich, high in fiber, vitamins, minerals, and antioxidants.

Nutritional values (per serving)

✓ Calories: 350-450
✓ Protein: 15-20g

- ✓ Fat: 15-20g
- ✓ Carbohydrates: 30-35g
- ✓ Fiber: 10-15g

Mushroom and Lentil Stuffed Bell Peppers

Ingredients:

Bell peppers, lentils, mushrooms, onion, garlic, vegetable broth, diced tomatoes, spinach, thyme, oregano, salt, pepper.

Instructions:

Sauté chopped mushrooms, onion, and garlic until softened. Stir in cooked lentils, diced tomatoes, spinach, thyme, oregano, salt, and pepper. Stuff mixture into halved bell peppers. Bake until peppers are tender.

Nutrients:

High in protein, fiber, vitamins, minerals, and antioxidants.

- ✓ Calories: 300-400
- ✓ Protein: 15-20g
- ✓ Fat: 5-10g
- ✓ Carbohydrates: 40-50g
- ✓ Fiber:15-20g

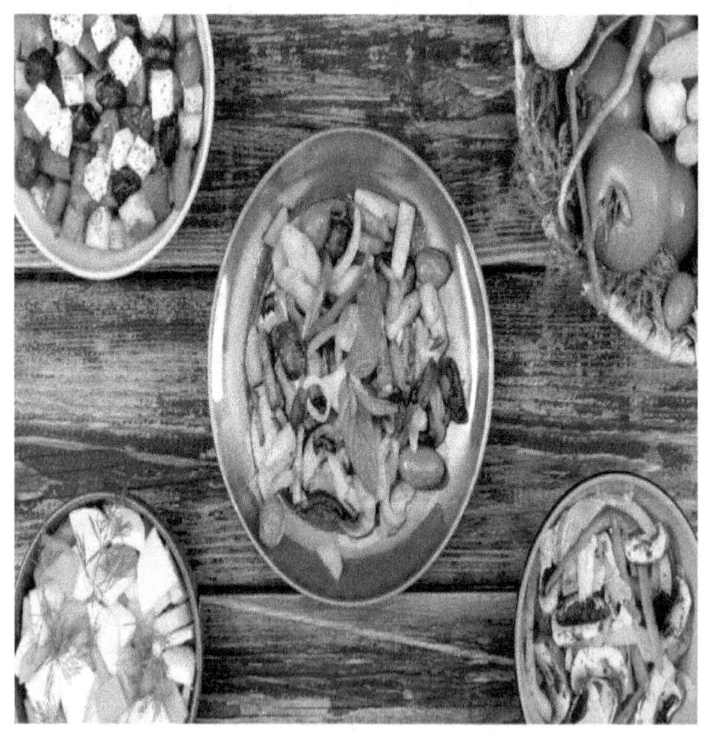

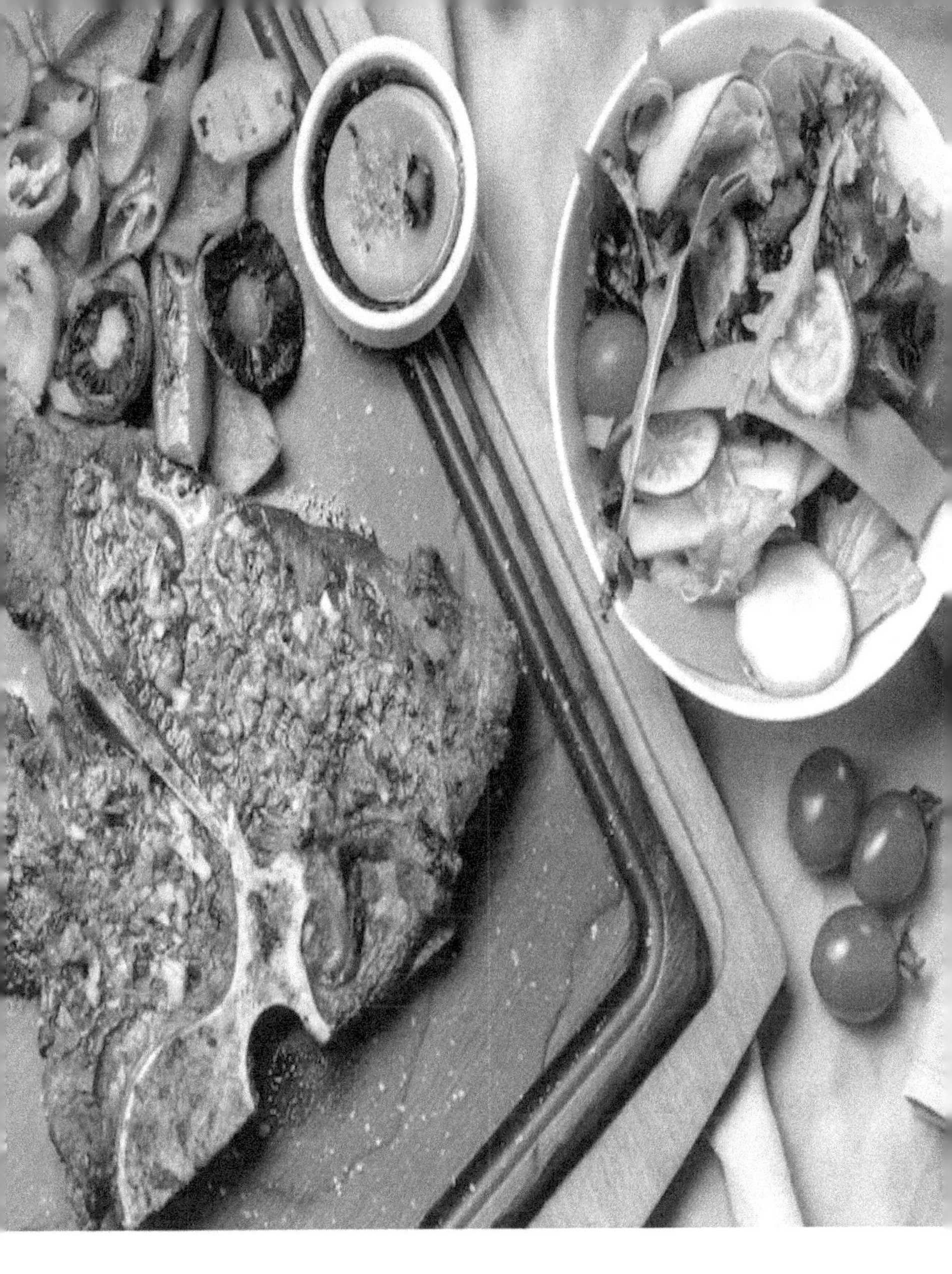

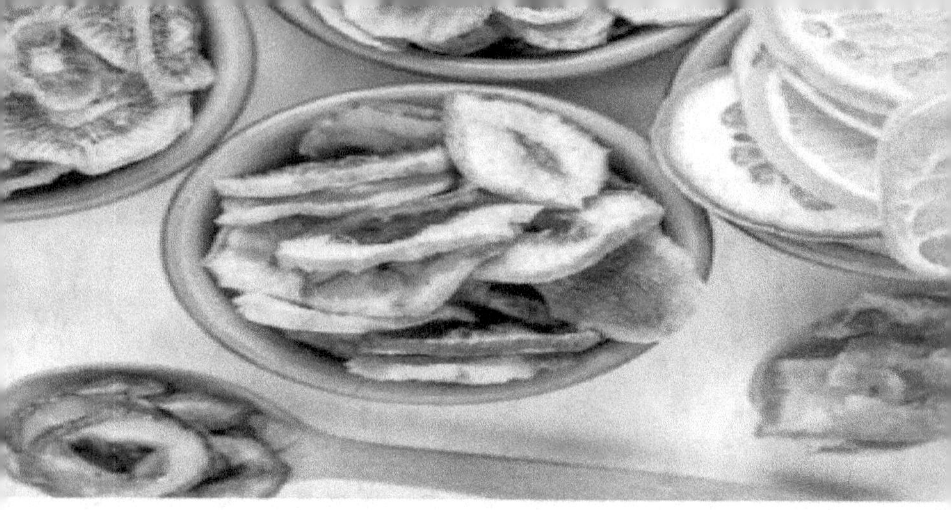

CHAPTER 6: SNACKS AND SIDES TO BOOST LIVER HEALTH

Greek Yogurt with Berries and Almonds

Ingredients:

Greek yogurt, mixed berries, almonds.

Instructions:

Serve Greek yogurt topped with mixed berries and sliced almonds.

Nutrients:

High in protein, fiber, vitamins, minerals, and antioxidants.

Nutritional Values (per serving)

- ✓ Calories: 200-250
- ✓ Protein: 15-20g
- ✓ Fat: 8-12g
- ✓ Carbohydrates: 20-25g
- ✓ Fiber: 5-8g

Vegetable Crudité with Hummus

Ingredients:

Carrot sticks, cucumber slices, bell pepper strips, cherry tomatoes, hummus.

Instructions:

Arrange vegetable sticks and slices on a plate. Serve with hummus for dipping.

Nutrients:

High in fiber, vitamins, minerals, and antioxidants.

Nutritional Values (per serving)

- ✓ Calories: 150-200
- ✓ Protein: 5-10g

- ✓ Fat: 8-12g
- ✓ Carbohydrates: 15-20g
- ✓ Fiber: 5-8g
- ✓ Baked Sweet Potato Fries

Ingredients:

Sweet potatoes, olive oil, paprika, garlic powder, salt.

Instructions:

Cut sweet potatoes into fries, toss with olive oil, paprika, garlic powder, and salt. Bake until crispy.

Nutrients:

High in fiber, vitamins, minerals, and antioxidants.

Nutritional Values (per serving)

- ✓ Calories: 150-200
- ✓ Protein: 2-4g
- ✓ Fat: 8-10g
- ✓ Carbohydrates: 20-25g
- ✓ Fiber: 3-5g

Avocado and Tomato Salad

Avocado, tomatoes, red onion, cilantro, lime juice, olive oil, salt, pepper.

Chop avocado and tomatoes, finely dice red onion, and chop cilantro. Toss together with lime juice, olive oil, salt, and pepper.

High in healthy fats, fiber, vitamins, minerals, and antioxidants.

- ✓ Calories: 150-200
- ✓ Protein: 2-4g
- ✓ Fat: 10-15g
- ✓ Carbohydrates: 10-15g
- ✓ Fiber: 5-8g

Edamame with Sea Salt

Ingredients:

Edamame (soybeans), sea salt.

Instructions:

Boil or steam edamame according to package instructions. Serve with a sprinkle of sea salt.

Nutrients:

High in protein, fiber, vitamins, minerals, and antioxidants.

Nutritional Values (per serving)

- ✓ Calories: 100-150
- ✓ Protein: 8-12g
- ✓ Fat: 3-5g
- ✓ Carbohydrates: 8-10g
- ✓ Fiber: 4-6g

Cucumber and Avocado Sushi Rolls

Ingredients:

Nori sheets, sushi rice, cucumber, avocado, rice vinegar, soy sauce, wasabi, pickled ginger.

Instructions:

Spread sushi rice on nori sheets, add sliced cucumber and avocado. Roll tightly, slice, and serve with soy sauce, wasabi, and pickled ginger.

Nutrients:

High in healthy fats, fiber, vitamins, minerals, and antioxidants.

Nutritional Values (per serving)

- ✓ Calories: 200-250
- ✓ Protein: 4-6g
- ✓ Fat: 8-10g
- ✓ Carbohydrates: 30-35g
- ✓ Fiber: 4-6g

Roasted Chickpeas

Ingredients:

Canned chickpeas, olive oil, cumin, paprika, garlic powder, salt.

Instructions:

Drain and rinse chickpeas, toss with olive oil, cumin, paprika, garlic powder, and salt. Roast until crispy.

Nutrients:

High in protein, fiber, vitamins, minerals, and antioxidants.

Nutritional Values (per serving)

- ✓ Calories: 150-200
- ✓ Protein: 6-8g
- ✓ Fat: 4-6g
- ✓ Carbohydrates: 20-25g
- ✓ Fiber: 6-8g

Spinach and Strawberry Salad

Ingredients:

Baby spinach, strawberries, goat cheese, balsamic vinegar, olive oil, honey, walnuts.

Instructions:

Toss baby spinach with sliced strawberries, crumbled goat cheese, balsamic vinegar, olive oil, and honey. Top with chopped walnuts.

Nutrients:

High in fiber, vitamins, minerals, and antioxidants.

Nutritional Values (per serving)

- ✓ Calories: 200-250
- ✓ Protein: 5-8g
- ✓ Fat: 10-15g
- ✓ Carbohydrates: 15-20g
- ✓ Fiber: 4-6g

Quinoa and Black Bean Salad

Ingredients:

Cooked quinoa, black beans, corn, bell peppers, red onion, cilantro, lime juice, olive oil, cumin, salt, pepper.

Instructions:

Mix cooked quinoa with black beans, corn, diced bell peppers, finely chopped red onion, and chopped cilantro. Dress with lime juice, olive oil, cumin, salt, and pepper.

Nutrients:

High in protein, fiber, vitamins, minerals, and antioxidants.

Nutritional Values (per serving)

- ✓ Calories: 250-300
- ✓ Protein: 8-10g
- ✓ Fat: 8-10g
- ✓ Carbohydrates: 35-40g

✓ Fiber: 6-8g

Roasted Beet and Goat Cheese Salad

Ingredients:

Roasted beets, mixed greens, goat cheese, walnuts, balsamic vinegar, olive oil, honey, salt, pepper.

Instructions:

Arrange roasted beets, mixed greens, crumbled goat cheese, and chopped walnuts on a plate. Dress with balsamic vinegar, olive oil, honey, salt, and pepper.

Nutrients:

High in fiber, vitamins, minerals, and antioxidants.

Nutritional Values (per serving)

✓ Calories: 200-250

✓ Protein: 6-8g

✓ Fat: 12-15g

✓ Carbohydrates: 15-20g

✓ Fiber: 5-8g

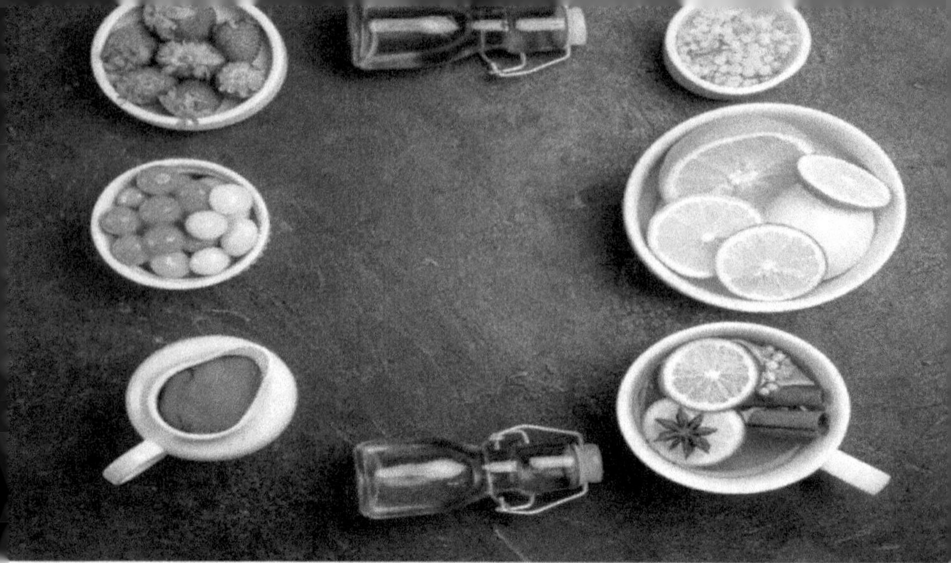

CHAPTER 7: BEVERAGES
FOR LIVER SUPPORT

Green Detox Smoothie

Ingredients:

Spinach, kale, cucumber, celery, green apple, lemon juice, ginger, water or coconut water.

Instructions:

Blend all ingredients until smooth.

Nutrients:

High in vitamins, minerals, antioxidants, and hydrating properties.

- ✓ Calories: 100-150
- ✓ Protein: 3-5g
- ✓ Fat: 1-2g
- ✓ Carbohydrates: 20-25g
- ✓ Fiber: 5-8g

Turmeric Ginger Tea

Ingredients:

Fresh turmeric root, fresh ginger root, water, honey (optional).

Instructions:

Grate turmeric and ginger roots into a saucepan, add water, and simmer for 10-15 minutes. Strain and sweeten with honey if desired.

Nutrients:

Contains anti-inflammatory compounds and antioxidants.

Nutritional Values (per serving)

- ✓ Calories: 10-20
- ✓ Protein: <1g
- ✓ Fat: <1g
- ✓ Carbohydrates: 2-5g
- ✓ Fiber: <1g

Beetroot Juice

Ingredients:

Fresh beets, carrots, apples, ginger (optional).

Instructions:

Run all ingredients through a juicer. Strain if desired.

Nutrients:

Rich in antioxidants, vitamins, and minerals, including betalains which support liver detoxification.

Nutritional Values (per serving)

- ✓ Calories: 100-150
- ✓ Protein: 2-4g

✓ Fat: <1g

✓ Carbohydrates: 25-30g

✓ Fiber: 3-5g

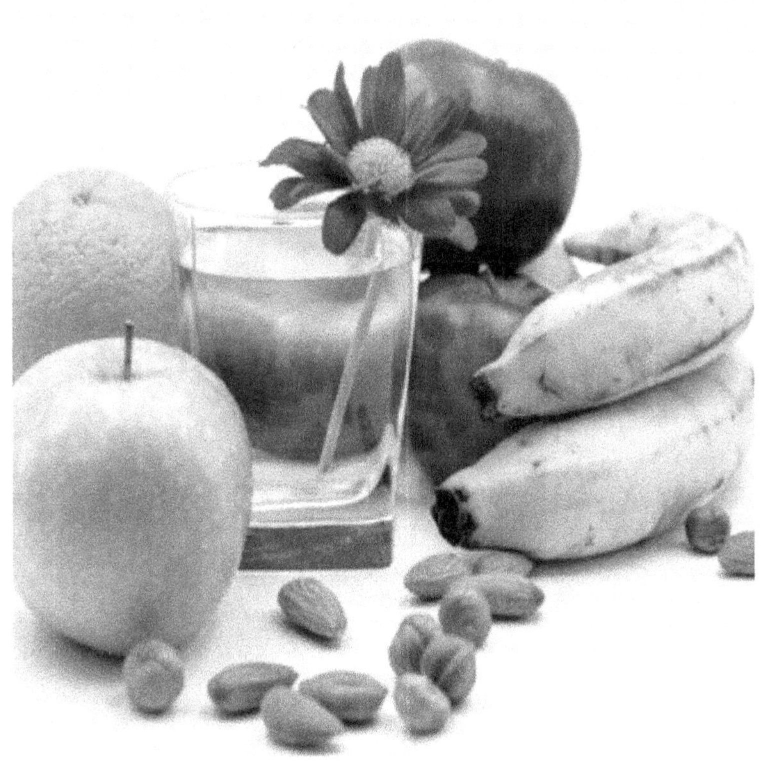

Dandelion Root Tea

Dandelion root tea bags or dried dandelion root, hot water.

Instructions:

Steep dandelion root tea bags or dried dandelion root in hot water for 5-10 minutes.

Nutrients:

Supports liver function and digestion.

Nutritional Values (per serving)

- ✓ Calories: 0
- ✓ Protein: 0g
- ✓ Fat: 0g
- ✓ Carbohydrates: 0g
- ✓ Fiber: 0g

Lemon Water

Fresh lemon juice, water, ice cubes.

Squeeze fresh lemon juice into water, add ice cubes
if desired.

Supports hydration and provides vitamin C, which
aids liver detoxification.

Nutritional Values (per serving)

- ✓ Calories: 5-10
- ✓ Protein: <1g
- ✓ Fat: <1g
- ✓ Carbohydrates: 2-5g
- ✓ Fiber: <1g

Minty Cucumber Lime Cooler

Cucumber, lime, mint leaves, water, ice cubes.

Blend cucumber, lime juice, mint leaves, and water until smooth. Serve over ice.

Hydrating, refreshing, and rich in vitamins and antioxidants.

- ✓ Calories: 20-30
- ✓ Protein: <1g
- ✓ Fat: <1g
- ✓ Carbohydrates: 5-10g
- ✓ Fiber: 1-2g

Ginger Lemon Detox Water

Ingredients:

Fresh ginger, lemon slices, water, ice cubes.

Instructions:

Infuse water with sliced ginger and lemon slices. Allow to sit for a few hours or overnight in the refrigerator. Serve chilled or over ice.

Nutrients:

Supports digestion, hydration, and liver detoxification.

Nutritional Values (per serving)

- ✓ Calories: 5-10
- ✓ Protein: <1g
- ✓ Fat: <1g
- ✓ Carbohydrates: 1-3g
- ✓ Fiber: <1g

Apple Cider Vinegar Tonic

Ingredients:

Apple cider vinegar, water, honey (optional).

Instructions:

Mix apple cider vinegar with water. Sweeten with honey if desired.

Nutrients:

Supports digestion and liver detoxification.

Nutritional Values (per serving)

- ✓ Calories: 5-10
- ✓ Protein: <1g
- ✓ Fat: <1g
- ✓ Carbohydrates: 1-3g
- ✓ Fiber: 0g

Matcha Green Tea

Matcha powder, hot water.

Whisk matcha powder into hot water until frothy.

Rich in antioxidants and catechins, which support liver health and detoxification.

Nutritional Values (per serving)

- ✓ Calories: 5-10
- ✓ Protein: <1g
- ✓ Fat: <1g
- ✓ Carbohydrates: <1g
- ✓ Fiber: <1g

Berry Blast Smoothie

Ingredients:

Mixed berries (such as strawberries, blueberries, raspberries), spinach, almond milk, chia seeds (optional), honey (optional).

Berry Blast Smoothie

Ingredients

1 cup mixed berries (strawberries, blueberries, raspberries)

1 banana

1/2 cup plain Greek yogurt

1/2 cup almond milk (or any milk of your choice)

1 tablespoon honey (optional)

Ice cubes (optional, for a colder smoothie)

Instructions

Wash the berries thoroughly under cold water and pat them dry.

Peel the banana and chop it into smaller chunks.

In a blender, combine the mixed berries, banana chunks, Greek yogurt, almond milk, and honey (if using).

Blend all the ingredients until smooth and creamy. If you prefer a thicker consistency, you can add more frozen berries or ice cubes.

Taste the smoothie and adjust sweetness if necessary by adding more honey.

Once the desired consistency and taste are achieved, pour the smoothie into glasses and serve immediately.

Nutritional Values (per serving, approximately)

- ✓ Calories: 150
- ✓ Total Fat: 1g
- ✓ Saturated Fat: 0g
- ✓ Cholesterol: 0mg
- ✓ Sodium: 50mg
- ✓ Total Carbohydrates: 32g

- ✓ Dietary Fiber: 5g
- ✓ Sugars: 21g
- ✓ Protein: 6g

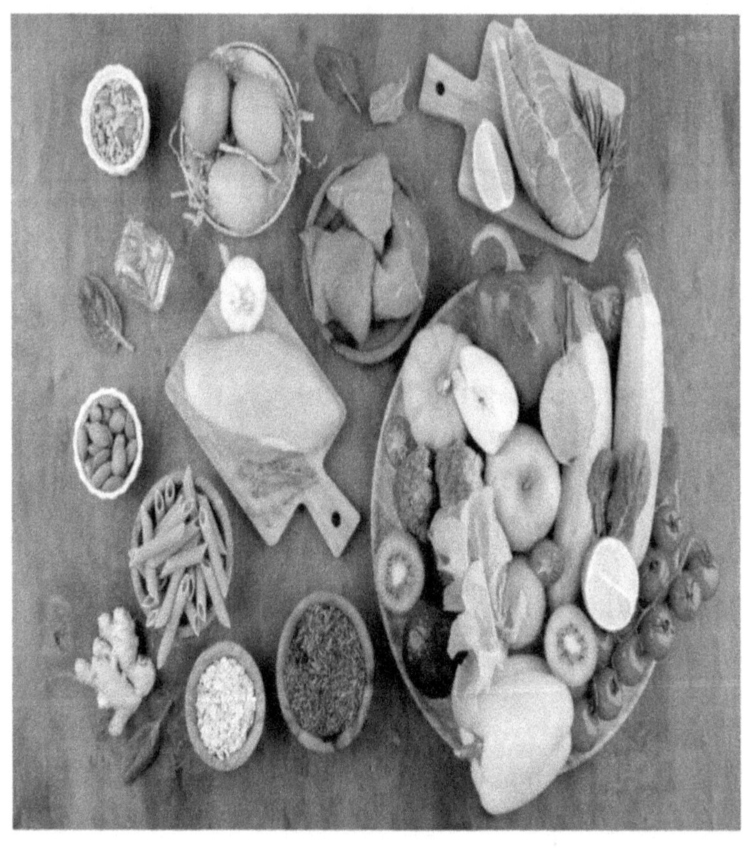

As you explore the recipes and insights within this cookbook, I kindly request a moment of your time. Your review on Amazon would greatly assist others on their journey to better liver health. Whether you found the recipes delicious, the nutritional tips valuable, or simply enjoyed the read, your feedback is invaluable. Thank you for considering sharing your thoughts and for being a part of spreading awareness about the importance of a healthy liver and balanced nutrition.

CONCLUSION

Encouragement for Continued Healthy Eating Habits

Every nutrient-dense decision you make today is a step toward a better, healthier tomorrow as you continue on your path to ideal liver health. Savor the mouthwatering tastes and wholesome components that promote your health, and acknowledge the strides you've already achieved. Every decision you make, whether it's enjoying a hearty supper with loved ones or beginning your day with a nutritious breakfast, moves you closer to your objectives. Remember that you're making an investment in your long-term health and vigor when you stick to your good eating habits. This is something you can handle.

In conclusion, it is both necessary and powerful to start the path to better liver health through mindful eating and healthy recipes. We've examined the complex relationship between diet and liver function in this fatty liver cookbook, which also provides a plethora of delectable recipes that promote liver health and general well-being. Every meal, from filling lunches to hearty feasts, has been thoughtfully developed to emphasize healthful ingredients and cooking methods that support liver heath. People can manage fatty liver disease and enhance their quality of life by adopting a diet high in fruits, vegetables, lean meats, whole grains, and healthy fats.

Beyond the recipes, however, is a deeper knowledge of fatty liver disease, including its causes, risk factors, and the significance of lifestyle changes for managing the condition. Equipped with expertise and gastronomic motivation, readers may make knowledgeable decisions, confidently maneuver through supermarket aisles, and set out on a path towards achieving optimal liver health. Let's take the knowledge and tastes from this cookbook with us as we turn the last page, knowing that every mouthful gets us one step closer to taking back control of our health and vitality. Cheers to fueling our bodies, nourishing our souls, and welcoming a future full of delectable opportunities.

www.ingramcontent.com/pod-product-compliance
Lightning Source LLC
Chambersburg PA
CBHW070823260726
48660CB00005B/1961